HABIT CHANGE

An Executive Coach's Step-by-Step Guide to Defeating Unwanted Behaviors

JEFF KAPLAN, PH.D.

ISBN-13: 978-0-9906529-1-5 (print)
ISBN-10: 0990652912 (print)

In order to receive additional copies of this book, contact:
Jeff Kaplan, <u>drjeff@drjeffkaplan.com</u>, 610.279.1408 (USA)

DEDICATION

This book is written with gratitude to all those who have entrusted me to help them improve their lives. You are my greatest teacher.

CONTENTS

Introduction

It's January 2: The New Year's resolutions have been made and it's time to get down to business! At the gym each machine has a line of new and eager but inexperienced members, clad in their brand new exercise attire, trying to navigate the unfamiliar equipment. Long-time clients, though impatiently waiting their turn, are soothed by the knowledge that this is a short-lived phenomenon. Within a week or two, most of the newbies will revert to the inertia that prompted them to resolve, "I will work out three times a week." Then all will be back to normal until next January 2!

Likewise, the latest diet books are flying off the shelves at the local bookstore or delivered (by drones?!) from the many online shopping sites. Every TV channel regularly blares, "You, too, can lose 50 lbs. in 3 weeks!" Marketers are definitely in on the secret! Once more, with hope triumphing over experience, the newly committed dieters have cleared the kitchen cupboards of all goodies and replaced them with rice cakes and other "healthy" snacks. Family members, now having to keep their fattening stash out of site, whisper to each other, "Don't worry, this will pass in a few weeks—or days!"

In my 30 years of helping people create sustained change, I have witnessed the above scenarios and those like them—promises to stop smoking, save money, slow down, spend more quality time with the family, develop a more positive attitude—play out over and over again. With each failure to sustain the habit change, the individual grows more and more frustrated and blames him or herself for a lack of willpower. Perhaps you can identify.

In this book, I have set down what I have found to be the guiding principles necessary for success in letting go of self-defeating habits and the specific practices that will put you on a path to creating and sustaining the changes you seek. They can be applied to your personal habits, your interpersonal relationships, and your interactions in the workplace. They include:

1. The causes of habit change failure

2. The role of self-awareness in creating sustained change

3. The limitation of willpower

4. The importance of intention vs. goal-setting

5. Setting an agenda

6. A formula to create and sustain change

7. Strategies to overcome common barriers to habit change

Chapter 1

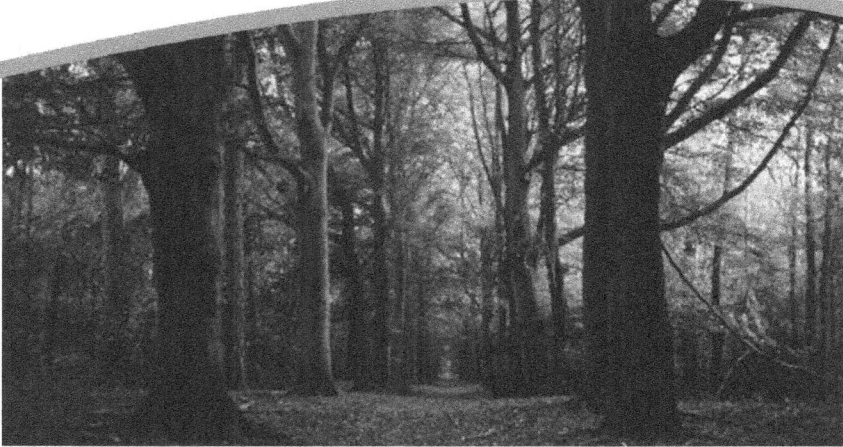

THE PATH IN THE WOODS

"As a single footstep will not make a path on the earth, so a single thought will not make a pathway in the mind."
Wilferd Arlan Peterson, 1900-1995

I HAVE NO WILLPOWER

If you ask a dozen people why they were unsuccessful in changing a habit or stopping a negative behavior, many of them might say they lack willpower. Tell someone that you've given up cigarettes or lost 30 pounds, and they'll tell you how much they admire your willpower. This belief is so widespread that most who fail over and over again to meet their habit change goals never consider any other explanation.

Consider Betty and Will:

Betty is a 52-year-old healthcare executive at an urban hospital. She has a loving family and good friends, and she feels fulfilled in her work. Yet, Betty is unhappy. Over the last 15 years, she has gradually gained weight, her stress has become almost unmanageable, her energy has decreased, and she has recently had trouble sleeping. She feels she always has to be "on" at her job, which is becoming increasingly complex in today's rapidly changing healthcare environment. Betty has unsuccessfully attempted several diets and exercise programs, but with the overwhelming number of compulsory morning and evening meetings, she just cannot find the time to eat well or exercise consistently. She began an 8-week yoga class, which she enjoyed, but attended only the first two classes— "something always gets in the way." Betty is perplexed. How is it that she truly believes she wants a healthy, fit body yet fails at each and every attempt to achieve her goal? Why, after losing five pounds, does she revert to the same behavior patterns that led her to gain weight in the first place? Why are her efforts so short-lived? "I just have no willpower," decides Betty.

Will is a 32-year-old attorney, a junior partner in a large law firm. His demanding job and never-ending efforts to climb the corporate ladder leave little time for his wife and two children. When he is home, he's in the den, door closed, totally absorbed in the computer screen in front of him. The family respects his privacy, accepting that his occupational demands often spill over into his private life, but wish that he could be more engaged in their activities. What they don't know and what Will himself has difficulty accepting is that he has become addicted to online gaming. The legal documents he brought home from the office sit untouched as he competes with other gamers to achieve the next level in the fast-moving video. What was originally a way to relax during his stressful final year in law school has progressed to an all-consuming obsession.He had convinced himself that gaming was a much-needed escape from his overwhelming workload. Now, though, he has to admit that his migraines, backaches, and recently-diagnosed carpal tunnel syndrome are directly related to his gaming. Frequent promises to himself to limit his time on the sites have been unsuccessful. Although he hasn't yet spent office time on gaming, he believes it's only a matter of time before he gives in to the compulsion to do so. Why would a professional like Will put at risk his job, his family, and his health for his addiction? And, why, in spite of his determined efforts, can't he find the willpower to stop?

CAUSE OF HABIT CHANGE FAILURE

Neuroscience, or "brain science"—not lack of willpower—explains why Betty and Will consistently fail to change their nutritional and exercise and gaming habits. Each time they repeat the negative behaviors, they strengthen certain neural pathways within their brains, reinforcing the likelihood of doing it again

To illustrate, consider a path in the woods created by people walking over the same route repeatedly. One person breaks virgin ground and walks from point A to point B, leaving only a small and possibly unnoticeable trail. Each time someone walks the exact same route, more brush gets pushed down, twigs and rocks get pushed or kicked aside, and a new pathway becomes more defined. This is what happens in the brain when the same behavior, be it negative or positive, is repeated again and again. Eventually, what was once a conscious thought is now a subconscious habit. Like the path in the woods, each attempt and failure solidifies the "failure to change" neuro-pathway in the brain, increasing the likelihood of future failures.

WILLPOWER IS UNSUSTAINABLE

Betty and Will, like 88% of people who attempt to create change or eliminate a negative habit, rely on willpower. This is unsuccessful because of the way our brains are wired.

The use of willpower requires activation of certain parts of the prefrontal cortex, the section of the brain responsible for making logical decisions. However, the prefrontal cortex takes a back seat when it comes to making choices on behaviors that have become habitual. In fact, by definition, there is no "choice" with habitual behavior. The prefrontal cortex is the area of higher brain functioning and, among other tasks, helps to regulate behavior using logical and rational thought processes. If changing a habit were the only object of focus for the prefrontal cortex, perhaps it would be possible to choose a new behavior that would immediately replace the negative one. But this is not the case. Throughout the day we make thousands of decisions and solve various problems. Many of the decisions we make are subconscious, such as brushing our teeth or getting dressed. Our brains are not wired to focus simultaneously on the hundreds and thousands of decisions we make daily. Another fact to consider is the prefrontal cortex becomes less active when one is under high levels of stress.

The following scenarios illustrate the process of a conscious act becoming a subconscious habit.

- You think about eating and make a deliberate act to do so; you then take a bite of food which is very much a conscious act. Your prefrontal cortex is in full swing, organizing the information coming in (such as previous knowledge about weight gain, how your peers perceive you at this moment, and the environment); analyzing the decision (weighing the pros and cons); and then taking "conscious action." Although eating certain foods may be a poor choice to the person who is dieting, it is a conscious choice.

  When you overeat, you subconsciously develop a negative habit; over time, overeating becomes less a conscious decision and more an automatic response to a subconscious desire. Certainly, the body's response to the sensory pleasures of food plays a part in "rewarding the behavior" and increasing the desire to eat.

- Exercise is similar. You are well aware of the tremendous benefits of exercise; however, you may lack the incentive to maintain a regular exercise routine. Perhaps you join a gym and hire a personal trainer. The trainer introduces you to the exercise equipment, classes, and routines to do at home, and even encourages you to start slow and set realistic goals based on your abilities and schedule. You leave the gym feeling proud of yourself and excited about the positive results you will gain by exercising. Yet, a week later, you cancel your follow-up appointment with the trainer. What happened? Despite a realistic goal, firm intention, and correct information, you fell back into old habits as a result of years of self-sabotaging, subconscious behaviors.

  Based on your history of starting and stopping exercise routines, you subconsciously go down the same "path in the woods" with the same negative results. You then mentally beat up on yourself for what you believe is a lack of willpower. A vicious cycle has formed, and you continue to undermine your desire to improve your health.

- This same scenario applies to interpersonal relationships. Perhaps you work with a disagreeable co-worker or boss. Repeated attempts at changing the dynamic between the two of you have been met only with failure. In spite of the best of intentions, your negative facial expression, tone of voice, and off-putting manner automatically arises as your "foe" approaches—displaying matching body language. These habit-forming behaviors have shaped your interaction. The game will continue until one of you comes to understand the dynamic at play and takes the initiative to acquire the knowledge and communication skills necessary to improve the relationship.

The following chapters will guide you in making positive changes in your life, help you become aware of subconscious behaviors that lead to poor behavioral choices, and help you understand the habit change process that can lead you down the path of success.

Chapter 2

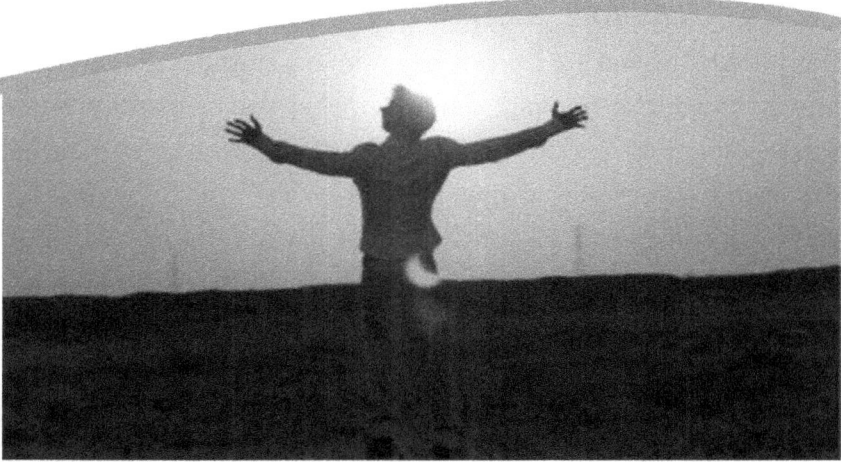

WAKING UP

*"No problem can be solved on the same
level of consciousness that created it."*
Albert Einstein, 1879-1995

Einstein understood that the secret to solving a problem is to first become more self-aware. To change our habits, we must first "wake up!" Our life today is the result of the infinite number of choices we've made each and every day. If we continue to make the same choices, consciously or unconsciously, we'll continue to get the same results.

BECOMING AWARE

The process of waking up can begin in any number of ways: You look in the mirror one day, don't like what you see, and promise yourself to enroll in a diet and fitness program; you recognize that you need to reassess your time priorities when your child asks why you never come to her Little League games; you come to realize that yelling and gesturing at the "idiotic" drivers on the road leaves you drained at the end of your commute and you decide to buy an audio book tape to engage your mind.

Usually, though, our negative habits are so much a part of our identity—"It's who I am"—that a more serious wake-up call is what finally gets our attention: Your drinking has resulted in a DUI or a serious accident; your spouse threatens to leave because of your verbal abuse; your unhealthy diet has resulted in a diagnosis of diabetes; you are faced with bankruptcy because of your over-spending.

Two motivators of change are "attraction" and "fear." Some of us are more attracted to the possibilities – "If I lose this weight, I'll look really good in my wedding dress," while others are more motivated by fear of the consequences of not changing – "If I don't stop eating this way, I could die and never see my grandchildren graduate." Whether you are motivated by attraction or fear may be situation-specific; yet, most of us tend to default to one or the other unless the reward (e.g., "Working hard will help us move into our dream house in a safe neighborhood.") or the price to pay (e.g., "If I don't stop I could lose my job and my marriage.") is very high.

LAYING THE GROUNDWORK

1. **Identify the true nature of the problem.** What often stands in the way of change is denial: The cause of my obesity is a glandular condition; I can't have an alcohol problem because I only drink beer; my hectic schedule gets in the way of my exercise program; I work hard and deserve to reward myself with luxuries once in a while.

2. **Recognize that willpower is not the answer.** Our daily lives are filled with distractions, some avoidable, others not. We learned in Chapter 1 that willpower is controlled by the part of the brain responsible for processing these distractions and making moment-to-moment decisions. Habits are unconscious behaviors that must be brought into conscious awareness to get the attention of, and a decision by, the prefrontal cortex.

3. **Take responsibility.** Blaming others for your behavior allows you to avoid recognizing the true nature of the problem and shirk taking responsibility for your actions: The host would be insulted if I refused the fattening dessert; I would be more productive at work if my boss treated me fairly; I would be more pleasant at home if the wife and kids kept the place neat. Putting yourself at the mercy of others keeps you a victim and takes away your power to control your own destiny.

4. **Understand that you cannot change anyone but yourself.** The belief that someone else is the cause of your problems often leads to an attempt to change that person rather than look inward. You can only change your attitude and your response

to others. Difficult interactions with people in your life can be dealt with by healthy boundary-setting, emotional detachment, and perhaps empathy in recognizing that they, too, may be dealing with difficult personal issues.

5. **Take a habit inventory.** You may have already decided on the glaring habit that you are eager to change—the one that causes you or others the most pain. As a matter of fact, the behavior may be so flagrant that you have developed a negative self-image and can see nothing good in yourself. A habit inventory will give you the opportunity to objectively acknowledge both your positive and your negative characteristics and habits. It's similar to a merchant checking the store shelves—what's good and stays, what's outdated and has to go, and what new items are needed. It will give you the proper perspective, enabling you to zero in on the behavior which will be the focus of your change process.

EXERCISE

In ten minutes, list as many of your behaviors as you can that support your physical, emotional or spiritual health (e.g., walk to work, eat breakfast, go to religious service, keep a gratitude journal). Be generous.

In ten minutes, list as many of your behaviors as you can that interfere with your physical, emotional or spiritual health (e.g., skipping meals, late bedtimes, shouting at a loved one). Focus on those behaviors that have the greatest negative impact.

6. **Ask for help.** You may find it difficult to accept that you cannot personally solve your own problems and think that asking for help is a sign of weakness. You may believe that turning to a professional or other resource will force you into decisions you are unprepared to make, or that you'll become someone unrecognizable to yourself. A professional will not do the work for you but can be a valuable resource in helping you achieve the change you seek.

BECOMING CONSCIOUS

Before embarking on the physical steps necessary for habit change, it will be necessary to prepare mentally—to move from subconscious to conscious thoughts and behaviors. The following two processes are effective means of accessing the area of the brain that will support your change efforts.

MINDFULNESS AND MEDITATION

Mindfulness is the practice of focusing one's attention on what is happening in the moment in a nonjudgmental way. For centuries, mindfulness meditation and other forms of mindfulness exercises have helped people gain greater clarity, make better choices, and even improve health and happiness.

Mindfulness meditation has its roots in East Asia and was brought to the United States in the early 1970s by Jack Kornfield, Joseph Goldstein, Sharon Salzberg and others. Jon Kabat-Zinn's eight-week, Mindfulness-Based Stress Reduction program also helped put this practice on the western map. Begun in 1979 at the University of Massachusetts Medical Center, it is now taught in nearly every US state and more than 30 countries. Hundreds of research articles have been published showing the benefits of mindfulness meditation—it reduces anxiety and depression, helps those with Attention Deficit Disorder, aids in developing compassion, and helps improve relationships.

Several companies have brought mindfulness training into the workplace because of its positive impact on performance, retention, customer service, and even bottom-line business results. These companies include AOL Time Warner, Apple, AstraZeneca, Deutsche Bank, Google, McKinsey, and Yahoo, to name a few. Mindfulness in the workplace has been shown to: improve work-related performance, enhance the ability to respond (rather than react) to situations, enhance self-management skill, improve concentration and mental focus, improve coping and stress management skills, increase self-esteem, increase energy, enhance the ability to relax and enjoy life and experience a greater sense of happiness. In this book, I refer to mindfulness as both a technique and a way of life.

Living mindfully means to live in the present moment—to speak, act and think with intention. It means to make decisions "consciously" rather than by default. For example:

- When speaking with someone mindfully, I am completely present with the person and seek to understand the meaning behind her words as opposed to being wrapped up in my thoughts with judgments ("I can't believe what an idiot this person is!") or waiting for the other person to take a breath so I can interject a thought I'm anxious to share.

- Eating mindfully is to be present with my food and the manner in which I eat. I take each bite, savoring the different colors and textures, aromas, and changing tastes in my mouth as the digestive enzymes in my saliva begin to break down the food as opposed to mindlessly eating while watching television, talking with someone, or driving from one appointment to the next.

• Acting mindfully is to be clear and focused on the purpose of my behaviors, keeping my head where my feet are, so to speak as opposed to hurrying from one task or appointment to the next, my mind jumping from topic to topic, and finding myself exhausted at the end of the day, wondering where my time has gone.

Mindfulness as a technique can take a number of forms. Teachers of mindfulness may train on specific practices, such as mindful eating, mindful walking, and mindful communication. We will limit our focus to mindfulness meditation. You will find specific instructions for a meditation practice in Chapter 5.

THREE QUESTION MANTRA

This is a technique I developed in my practice to help clients change unhealthy habits. It is a three-step commitment process designed to raise awareness and bring in-the-moment accountability.

A consistent meditation practice and regular use of the three question mantra can awaken the desire to make decisions that most markedly support physical, emotional, social, and spiritual health.

Chapter 3

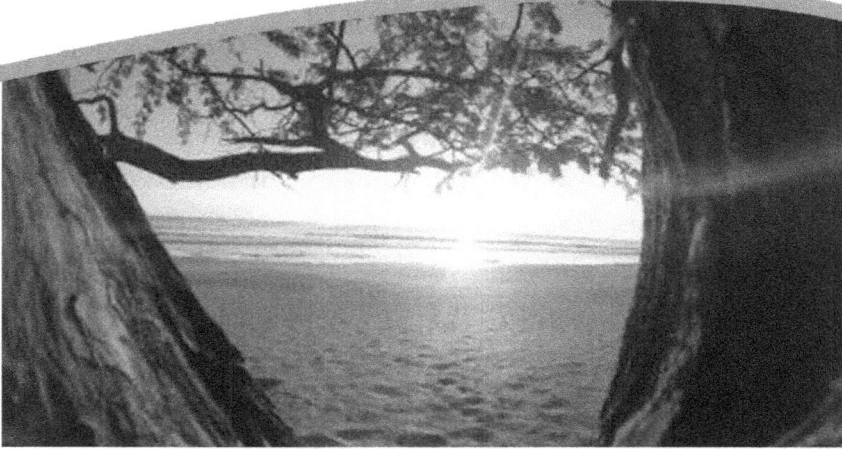

PREPARING FOR CHANGE

*"To solve a problem, it would be broken down
in a series of questions, the answers to which
gradually distill the answer a person would seek."*
Socrates, 470-399 BCE

DEVELOP AN ACTION PLAN

In the previous chapters, you learned (1) why willpower fails as a change agent when you're attempting to rid yourself of a deep-seated habit or negative behavior, (2) the critical role self-awareness plays in laying the groundwork for success, and (3) the importance of advancing the waking-up process with a daily mindfulness exercise and a habit inventory.

We'll assume that you have familiarized yourself with, and begun, the mindfulness exercises; taken an honest look at both your liabilities and your assets; and chosen the behavior you most want to change. Completing the following seven steps will help you to develop an effective action plan. Answering the questions and completing the suggested exercises will ensure that you have considered each aspect of your plan and are prepared to address any hurdle you might encounter as you go forward. Taking the time to thoroughly follow these steps is crucial to your habit change success.

STEP 1. OBTAIN ACCURATE INFORMATION

Whether the problem you wish to address is diet, exercise, smoking cessation, anger management, or workplace issues, you may think there could not possibly be anything more you need to know about it. However, there is a wealth of research data published regularly on any and every topic. You will find information on your issue on websites, television, and radio, and in social media, blogs, organizational journals, newspapers, and magazines. You may be surprised at what you discover and find it helpful in clarifying your goal and setting your action steps. Just be sure to limit your search to known and trusted sources.

- *Have you researched your intended goal and confirmed that you have the latest data?*

- *Have you obtained your information from reliable sources?*

- *Have you made assumptions about any of the information you have?*

EXERCISE

Conduct an internet search on the goal you've selected. Note the variety of options and select several sites published by reputable associations and organizations. Make note of any new or pertinent information. Bookmark the sites for future reference.

STEP 2: SET CLEARLY-DEFINED AND MEASURABLE GOALS

If you have obtained sufficient information and made a decision on a particular habit you wish to change, it's time to lay out your action plan. Success will require a REAL (realistic, evaluative, action-oriented, limited) goal. This will be discussed in detail in Chapter 5. Your action steps must be precise and easily measurable.

- *Is your goal well-thought out and consistent with your abilities?*

- *Are the action steps, time commitments, and assessment factors realistic and appropriate for your stated goal?*

EXERCISE

Identify a specific and measurable goal (e.g., lose 10 pounds) and a specific and measurable action step (e.g., walk 5 min/day, 3 days/week for 2 weeks). Be sure to clearly define your goal and action step.

STEP 3.
SELECT ONLY GOALS TO WHICH YOU ARE FIRMLY COMMITTED

Consider all the implications of pursuing and achieving your goal. Going into it with "eyes wide open" will help to avoid being taken off purpose by an unanticipated consequence of your action steps. Visualizing the rewards of achieving your goal can increase enthusiasm and minimize the chance of your failing into the "victim role" because of any sacrifices required of you. Also, remember that to be successful no one can want change more for you than you want it for yourself.

- *What sacrifices will be necessary to achieve my goal?*

- *How can I become more enthusiastic about pursuing this goal?*

- *Would a smaller or larger goal provide more motivation?*

- *What will be possible if I achieve my goal? How can I keep this in the forefront of my mind throughout the day?*

- *How will achieving this goal both positively and negatively impact my life? How can I maximize the positive and minimize the negative?*

- *Am I firmly committed to this goal or is it one I feel I "should" pursue or one that others want for me?*

EXERCISE

Using the goal you previously identified, select three clear, specific, SMALL action steps by asking yourself: (1) What will help me reach my goal? (2) What am I actually willing to do? (3) How will this positively and/or negatively impact my life? (4) What supports can I put in place to ensure success with each step? Commit only to the steps you are confident of taking.

STEP 4:
BUILD CONFIDENCE IN YOUR ABILITY TO CREATE CHANGE

Perhaps after having tried and failed on numerous occasions to break yourself of an unwanted habit you've developed a "failure mentality." The negative self-talk this produces is a significant barrier to success. Mindfulness exercises are valuable tools to help you develop a more positive attitude and outlook. They will enable you to substitute positive thoughts for negative ones and to visualize yourself successfully achieving your goal.

Selecting a large-scale goal, such as "live a more healthy lifestyle," which encompasses so many aspects of day-to-day living, is a set-up for failure. Meeting smaller, more achievable goals will improve your self-confidence and provide a foundation upon which to build future successes.

- *What positive thought will I substitute when memories of previous failed attempts at achieving this goal creep in?*

- *What tools will help me to frequently visualize myself achieving this goal?*

- *How can I break down my goal into several smaller steps?*

EXERCISE

In 12 words or short phrases, describe yourself in relation to your goal. For example, if your goal is to be a better listener, descriptors might include: bottom liner, tactless, fixer, insensitive. Now list their opposites—the words you expect will describe you once you've met your goal: open-minded, thoughtful, perceptive, understanding.

STEP 5. ACQUIRE NECESSARY EXTERNAL RESOURCES & ENLIST COMMUNITY SUPPORT

Although you cannot depend on others for your success, gaining the support of your family and others close to you will do much to aid in carrying out your action plan. Reviewing your own resources—money, time, energy, etc.—will be necessary to ensure that your plan is feasible. There is no guarantee that these will not change as you put your plan into action, but once you've investigated each of the factors, you'll be better able to adjust more easily to new circumstances, should they arise. Using the three step mantra introduced in Chapter 2 and described with more detail in Chapter 5 will help you keep your goal in the forefront of your mind.

- *Do I have the financial and public support necessary to achieve my goal?*

- *Have I made time allowances in my schedule to execute my action plan?*

- *Have I reviewed environmental factors (distances, locations) that could impact my action plan?*

- *Did I solicit the support of those who, intentionally or unintentionally, may attempt to sabotage my efforts at change; do I need to set boundaries?*

- *What structures have I created (reminders) to keep my goal in the forefront of my mind?*

EXERCISE

Based on your identified goal, list the resources and supports you will need to help ensure your success. Then separate them into two lists — "Must have" and "Would like to have."

STEP 6. ADDRESS MEDICAL OR PSYCHOLOGICAL ISSUES

Pick up a bottle of vitamins or an over-the-counter medication and you will see on the label words to the effect, "Before using, check with your physician." If you sign up for membership at a gym, you will be advised to obtain a medical clearance if you have a condition which could be negatively impacted by certain exercises. The same precaution should apply before you undertake any habit change that could affect your physical, mental, or emotional health. If you are under treatment for a medical or mental health condition, you should discuss any planned changes to your normal schedule or practices with your health care provider. In addition to giving you important information, they can be a valuable source of support as you pursue your goal.

- *Does my goal and action plan take into consideration any physical limitations I may have?*

- *If I suffer from a medical or health-related issue and my goal involves diet, exercise, or other such activity, have I obtained clearance from my physician or other medical provider?*

- *If I am under the treatment of a psychiatrist, psychotherapist, or other mental health practitioner, have I discussed my intended goal and action steps to be sure they will not interfere with my course of treatment?*

- *Have I discussed with my prescriber any medications or other substances I take, which could affect my energy, endurance, or sense of balance, as they may relate to my goal and action steps?*

EXERCISE

Schedule an appointment or a telephone consultation with your health care providers to discuss with them, and obtain their concurrence on, your specific goal and action steps.

STEP 7. RESOLVE VALUES CONFLICTS

Although a goal may be desirable, if it and/or your action steps interfere with a closely held value, the value will win every time. For example, if your exercise schedule takes you away from important family activities, you will likely choose your family over the workout. A values conflict doesn't necessarily mean that you will have to abandon your goal completely. An alternative would be to modify your goal or action steps to avoid the conflict.

- *Is the way in which I am attempting to achieve my goal interfering with a more important/equally important value?*

- *What values may be in conflict?*

- *Have I considered what I may need to say "no" to in order to create success; what I may need to say "yes" to?*

- *Can I formulate a plan to resolve the conflict, honoring each of my values?*

EXERCISE

Write a list of your top 10 values and place them in order from most important to least important. (You can find a list of over 350 values on the internet). You may want to check with those who know you well to see if they agree with the values you've chosen as your top 10. Sometimes it can be difficult to discern between values that are truly at the core of your being versus values you believe "should" be at the core of your being. Also, be sure that any action steps you've already identified or will create are aligned with these values. For those that do not, modify the action step so that it does not interfere with a top value.

Chapter 4

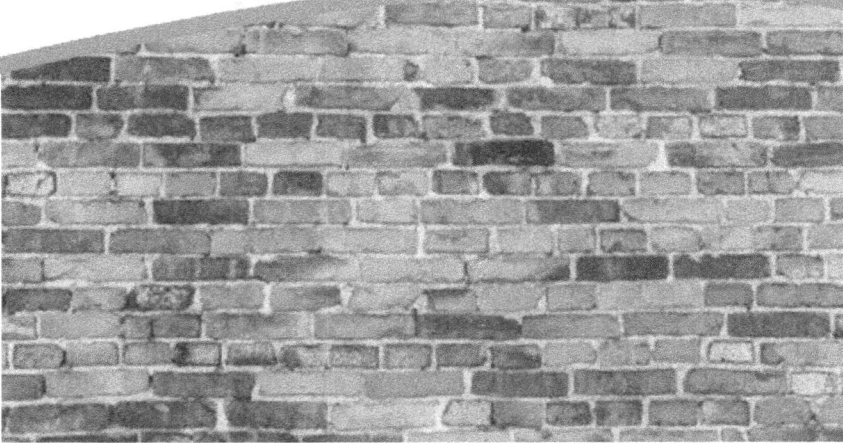

BARRIERS TO CHANGE

"New ideas are not only the enemies of old ones;
they also appear often in an extremely unacceptable form."
Carl Gustav Jung, 1875-1961

Attempts to create any significant habit change will most likely be met with internal resistance and may arise at the beginning of, or at any time during, the change process. Experience with clients in my practice over many years has shown that resistance usually exhibits as one or more of the seven barriers detailed in this chapter. You will note that they correspond to the seven action steps covered in Chapter 3. Reviewing the questions associated with your action steps can help you identify and address any resistance you encounter. Although you may experience a range of emotions when a barrier surfaces, it can often be identified by one particular feeling. Recognizing and addressing a barrier as soon as it surfaces is critical to your success. Failure to do so can result in a downward spiral and possible abandonment of your goal.

Common Barriers to Change	Associated Feeling
Lack of information	Confusion
Lack of clearly-defined goals	Discouragement
Lack of motivation	Apathy
Lack of confidence	Fear
Lack of external resources and support	Anger
Medical or psychological issues	Discontentment
Values conflict	Frustration

RESISTANCE TO CHANGE

As we learned earlier, our ways of behaving are deeply ingrained and directly linked to the vision we have of ourselves. There is much physical, emotional, and environmental underpinning supporting our actions. Think of the last time you attempted and failed to eliminate a negative habit (overeating, speaking harshly to a loved one, procrastinating) or acquire a positive one (regular exercise, daily meditation, timeliness). What was it that got in your way? A typical response might be: "Not enough time," "I was distracted," "I couldn't stick with it," or "I got lazy." The reason is actually much more complicated, as the following example illustrates:

• You have made repeated attempts to adhere to a healthy diet/ exercise program and consistently failed, often in spite of initial progress. What you don't realize is that much is going on within and around supporting the image of yourself as overweight. Your beliefs, thoughts, and actions are those of an overweight person. Perhaps you were raised in a household where it was unacceptable not to eat all the food served to you; you've become friends with your favorite sales associate at the Big and Tall clothing store; you're surrounded by overweight friends and family members; you habitually select the same foods from the grocery store aisles and frequent the same restaurants or fast food eateries; you avoid using a body-weight scale; you avoid certain places, people, or conversations because you're embarrassed about your weight; you have regular conversations with your physician about health problems related to being overweight; you purchase cars based on the driver's seat design; you see yourself as a failure when it comes to losing weight.

Thus, what might seem like a simple task (e.g., eat healthier and exercise) is actually an attempt to infiltrate an entire system of thoughts, feelings, and behaviors associated with being overweight. Attempting to change the outcome, i.e., lose weight, is going to be met with resistance from the entire system. Initial actions, such as one week of avoiding sweets, will be like a rubber band stretched until it can stretch no more without breaking. Once the rubber band is released, you will travel the path of least resistance, reverting to your former state, only a little more worn. Had you understood the pitfalls you might encounter and made the necessary preparations prior to embarking on your change journey, you would have had ready strategies to overcome an obstacle as it arose.

OVERCOMING BARRIERS

Following are scenarios to illustrate how each barrier may exhibit and suggestions on how it can be overcome. These examples may not reflect your particular situation; they are simply meant to illustrate how failing to consider each step thoroughly could thwart your goal.

1. **Lack of Information**

    Failure to obtain accurate information or to assume that the information you already have is correct can derail your progress.

    *   Imagine that you've taken your family to dinner to celebrate a member's birthday. You were quite embarrassed when the server notified you that your credit card had been refused. This was the last of your six cards, all now maxed out. Also, you've begun to receive nasty calls from bill collectors. You finally admit that your spending is out of control and vow to do something about it. You find an online debt consolidation company that promises to clear up your debt within 24 months and repair your credit. You are advised against filing for bankruptcy. As requested, you submitted all of your bills and your bank account information, with the company's assurance that each of your creditors was contacted and a payment plan arranged. The payments would be electronically transferred from your checking account. Next, you overnight the company's upfront fee of $1,000. Not surprisingly, within a short time you begin to receive calls from bill collectors—although the money has been disappearing from your bank account, the bills have not been paid. What happened?

        Had you conducted an online search of "debt consolidation" and "credit card repair," you would have learned that these are popular areas for scammers. Although there are many reputable companies providing financial services, fraudulent groups operating both in and outside the country can advertise online and ensnare vulnerable individuals desperate to resolve their financial issues. The Federal Trade Commission is an excellent resource for up-do-date information on dealing with debt. OnGuardOnline.gov publishes information on known scams and how to avoid them. Also, many communities and nonprofit organizations provide credit counseling services at no charge or for a small fee.

- Consider that your job-related goal is to be promoted to a supervisory position in your company within two years. In an effort to gain the attention of upper level management, you volunteer for a high-visibility project which you believe will prove your value to the organization. You are given the assignment and only after studying it carefully do you realize that adding the multiple tasks required of it to your already heavy workload will make it impossible to meet the milestones set for the project. Also, you will need to research certain elements of the task with which you are unfamiliar. Not wanting to admit that you're not up to the task, you labor long hours but soon have to admit that you will be unable to meet the deadline. The attention you gain from upper management is not positive and could derail your future opportunities with the company.

How did your good intention end in such failure? Your eagerness to get ahead led you to short-change your first action step and make a commitment for which you were not prepared. Had you thoroughly investigated the project's components and requirements before volunteering for it and taken into consideration the extent to which it would compete with your already heavy workload, you would have realized that you were "biting off more than you could chew." With full knowledge of the magnitude of the project, you may have decided against volunteering; asked about the possibility of a time extension; or, instead of taking on the entire project yourself, formed a team to share the tasks and rearranged your schedule to accommodate the additional duties.

2. **Lack of Clearly-defined and Measurable Goals**
Vague or hastily set goals and/or unclear measurement factors will ultimately lead to discouragement and most likely abandonment of your action plan.

- Assume it's Saturday night and you're exhausted after a day of holiday shopping. You've worked out twice this week and only have one more 30-minute session to honor your three-times-per-week exercise commitment. Getting on the treadmill in your exhausted state is the last thing you want to do tonight, and tomorrow will be a busy day getting the house ready for a party, grocery shopping, and wrapping gifts. For a moment, you're disheartened, realizing you either have to work out or dishonor your commitment. Then the light bulb goes off. "I've walked at least 30 minutes with all the running around I did today at the shopping malls." The relief pours through your body. "Whew...avoided that problem."

But did you really? What just happened is you bargained with yourself. Using this as justification, "working out 30 minutes" can now mean almost anything you want it to. And, while you can temporarily fool yourself into thinking you're off the hook, your mind knows better. Like the one loose thread you pull from a knitted sweater, this action becomes the beginning of the end and the plan is ruined. Very shortly thereafter, you become discouraged over your failure to make progress and stop exercising altogether.

Why did this happen? Your action step was not explicit or clearly defined. "Exercise three times a week" was vague and, like a good lawyer, you found a loophole—one that would serve you temporarily but would be the beginning of the end of honoring your commitment. What could have been the solution? Vowing to walk on the treadmill for 30 minutes on Monday, Wednesday, and Friday, would have closed the loophole. By Saturday, you would have met your goal and not had another session facing you when you were already over-committed.

• Vague goal-setting in the workplace can result in confusion, loss of revenue, waste of resources, and unmet obligations. As a supervisor, giving employees instructions on the run, while your mind is on another matter, or without confirming that the goal and necessary actions steps are clearly understood, is a setup for failure. In some cultures, it is considered disrespectful to question a supervisor; such a staffer will do the best he can with what he assumes is the assigned task. To ensure that the goals were clearly-defined and measurable, you would have followed up verbal instructions with a written confirmation of the assignment, milestones, and completion date.

3. **Lack of Motivation**

Lack of motivation is one of the top two reasons people fail to follow through on their action plan (the other is lack of confidence). Failure to understand your "motivational boundaries" can lead you to make commitments "you should" or ones you make blindly.

- Let's say that you look in the mirror one day and are unhappy with how much weight you've gained over the holidays. You feel motivated to lose the extra pounds. In reality, though, you want the weight to be reduced, but are you really motivated to change the behavior that led to this result in the first place? At the urging of your spouse, you agree to an eating and exercise program. When eating the healthy meals she prepares at home, guilt wells up when you recall your outside-the-home fare. On workdays, you regularly have lunch with several coworkers and frequent the nearby fast-food eatery. Despite good intentions, you continue to pass up the salads and other healthy menu options for the double bacon cheeseburger with fries. And, try as you might, you can't resist the homemade sweets that show up regularly in the break room. After a long day at work and the post-lunch slump, you say you're "too lazy" to go to the gym, not realizing that the negative self-talk is disempowering and presumes some inherent unchangeable trait. A more constructive approach is to consider the power of motivation.

Imagine that you will be given $100 million of tax-free money and ensured eternal happiness for you and your family if you adhere to your eating plan and go to the gym six times over the course of a two-week period. Will you be "lazy" then or will you figure out a way to comply? Obviously, you will need a more realistic motivator: No need to spend money on larger clothes; have more energy; limit health care costs; be free of guilt; look in the mirror without wincing! To reinforce your commitment, you pledge to donate $10 to a cause you abhor each time you fail to honor your commitment. As an added stimulus, you keep within easy reach a photo of yourself at your fittest to remind you of "what is possible!"

• Low motivation was the issue for a client of mine who works for a large global organization. He would often use his travel schedule as the excuse for failure to manage his diet. Yes, eating healthily can be more challenging when one is on the road and/or when most meals are taken as a guest in settings in which it would seem rude to reject the food offered.

Our work together enabled him to see how allowing this to be a barrier, rather than a challenge to overcome, was to surrender his power to impact the change he sought. If he were gravely allergic to the foods being served, he would figure out a way both to do his job and stay healthy. Once this executive was ready to take full responsibility and stop hiding behind excuses, he began a nutritional process that led to a 50-pound weight loss in less than nine months.

When planning action steps toward a particular outcome, there is no guarantee you will reach your goal—and all that sacrifice may be for naught. Imagine the difference between a great authority figure guaranteeing that if you take a set of specific action steps you will undoubtedly achieve the results you seek versus the more uncertain world we actually live in where there are no hard and fast guarantees. Thus, when it comes to motivation, you must: (1) first truly understand the sacrifices and impact of setting the goal you seek to achieve; (2) be willing to make the sacrifices, understanding the choice to do so is yours; and (3) be so fully committed to the process that you're willing to go forward with the necessary sacrifices without a guarantee of success.

4. **Lack of Confidence**

Lack of confidence is the other top barrier to change. Not believing in oneself or being unable to see oneself achieving a desired goal will impede progress. Repeated half-hearted, unsuccessful attempts to change an unwanted behavior—be it overeating, smoking, procrastination, negative thinking—results in a "failure self-image." The negative self-talk which follows—"Why do I even try?" "I have no willpower." "Nothing I do ever works out."—reinforces the negative self-image, making it increasingly more difficult to achieve the desired outcome. Lack of confidence may exhibit in diverse and sometimes seemingly paradoxical ways.

• Sharon sought help with her lack of self-confidence because she feared it could result in social isolation and loss of important friendships. She had avoided repaying the numerous generous friends who entertained her at their homes over the last several years due to her fear of "not meeting their standards." Being somewhat of a perfectionist, she thought that inviting people to her home for a dinner party required her to prepare a meal of 5-star quality. The negative self-talk, "I'm a terrible cook," and the belief that everyone else is a top chef provided an excuse for inaction. It didn't help that each time she considered issuing an invitation, what came to mind was the disastrous dinner she prepared years ago for her daughter's fiancé and his parents for a "get to know you" before the wedding. The roast and vegetables were under-cooked, the mashed potatoes and gravy were lumpy, and the mushroom dish was unrecognizable! And she was so stressed and exhausted that she couldn't enjoy the company.

Sharon came to realize that the most important aspect of any social event is the interaction with friends. She admitted that the alternative to entertaining, continuing to let the invitations pile up, would be a source of increasing stress and self-doubt and could result in a reluctance to accept future invitations and risk distancing herself from good friends. She set a goal to begin to repay her friends at a comfortable schedule. Instead of poring over cookbooks and preparing everything from scratch, she discovered a number of low-stress options for entertaining: a theme dinner—Mexican, Chinese, pizza party—with prepared foods purchased from a local restaurant or market; celebrate a holiday open house with simple finger foods; over time, invitation individuals or small groups of friends to be her guests at a restaurant.

- Picture yourself as a highly-skilled employee whose goal is to advance in your career. On paper you have all the qualifications to rise to the top of your organization. However, your lack of confidence prevents you from assuming a lead role in high-visibility projects and actively participating in meetings and conferences. The self-talk here might be, "I'm not good enough," "They really don't want to hear what I have to say," "I might make a fool of myself." Substituting an affirmative thought when a negative one creeps in; e.g., "I know as much about this subject as the others in this meeting and have something of value to contribute." In this case, your action plan may include participation in a group such as Toastmasters to help you overcome the fear of speaking to a group.

Conversely, a colleague who is considered by others to be overly self-confident—often interrupting a speaker, interjecting his own comments out of turn, jumping to erroneous conclusions because he failed to pay attention to the information presented—may also suffer from lack of confidence and a negative self-image with a constant need to prove himself "as good as." This over-zealous person's action plan may include a commitment to listen attentively when others are speaking and holding one's comments until the other speaker is through.

Lack of confidence is one of the principal barriers to workplace success. It prevents leaders (and would-be leaders) from seeking the help they need because of a fear of being "found out"). It also limits creativity and interferes with risk-taking. Resources within organizations to help employees with these concerns may include Employee Assistance Programs (EAP), which offer confidential counseling and referral services to address both personal and work-related issues, and executive coaching to aid their staff in addressing personal and job-related barriers to reach their greatest potential.

Overcoming a lack of self-confidence probably will not happen overnight and may require professional help. However, if you have taken a thorough habit inventory, you will have acknowledged your positive attributes as well as your negative ones and, hopefully, gained a more balanced self-image. The mindfulness exercises outlined in this book also can assist in overcoming lack of confidence.

5. Lack of External Resources and Support

Because our day-to-day decisions are influenced by innumerable internal and external factors, our physical environment and the people in our lives play a key role when we are attempting a significant change or striving to achieve a specific goal.

- Imagine that you are attempting to eat healthier and exercise as two parts of an overall plan to lose excess body fat. Despite promises to do so, family members have not kept cookies, chips, and other comfort foods out of the kitchen. Annoyance arises in you each time you encounter one of the forbidden foods. If the cupboards were free of these items, you would have to make a concerted effort to drive to the store to acquire them; having them within easy reach is too much of a temptation. A solution may be to ask your family to keep their snacks in one closet that you can easily avoid. To remind yourself that the closet is a danger zone for you, you might tape a skull and crossbones symbol to the closet door.

- With regard to exercise, let's assume that your goal is to work out for one hour, three times a week. Your house is too small for a treadmill or other exercise equipment. Your budget does not currently allow for membership in the nearby gym. The YMCA is affordable but it's a 30-minute drive from your house and in the opposite direction from your workplace. How often do you think you will decide to forego your workout, knowing it will take a total of three hours out of your already tight schedule?

  Rather than fret over the obstacles, you will need to look for alternatives to fit your financial and time constraints. Fitness and sports shops have an array of inexpensive exercise props—weights and dumbbells, balance balls, jump ropes, and resistance bands. Yoga classes are popping up in every neighborhood. Perhaps you have a friend with an in-home gym. Is there a walking trail near your home or a nearby mall (unless window shopping will slow down your pace!)? You might hire a fitness trainer for a few sessions to help you plan your exercise program and suggest incentives to keep you on track.

- Lack of external resources or support is another common barrier to success in the work environment. Limited capital, both human and financial; disengaged supervisors; a poorly-skilled workforce; and time constraints hamper a company's ability to carry out its mission.

From an organizational standpoint, success within these limitations requires (1) strong leadership to set clear goals and priorities, especially where there are competing demands; (2) an effective management team to assign tasks which support the mission and set achievable milestones; (3) unbiased supervision by rewarding high performers and giving honest feedback to poor performers, with a plan to bring work up to standards; (4) support of upper management when disciplinary action of an employee is necessary; (5) maintenance of a professional environment by addressing conduct issues.

Whatever your career goals, lack of resources and support will affect you to a greater or lesser extent. If you're in a managerial position, you will have responsibility for juggling these duties and demands with limited resources, as well as attempting to keep the staff energized and productive. If you're not at the top, and management is failing in its attempts to keep the organization on firm footing and support the staff, you may feel angry, disillusioned, and victimized.

Talk with your manager and/or HR Business Partner if you have concerns about your workplace and/or your role within it. If the situation seems too problematic, such as a work environment that is misaligned with your own personal and professional values, it may be time to explore other employment opportunities.

6. **Medical or Psychological Issues**

- Assume your physician has advised you to embark on a health regimen which is to include regular exercise and a reduction of calories in your diet. You commit to walk on a treadmill at a moderate pace for 30 minutes three times per week and adhere to the balanced diet he recommended. You honor your exercise commitment and Day 1 is a success. "That was easy," so the next time you decide to work out "harder;" over the following weeks you continue to increase your pace and time. By the third week, you notice that your clothes are fitting a little looser. Again you increase both your speed and time, working up a good sweat for nearly an hour. You also decide to modify the diet you were given and eliminate all carbs, hoping to speed up your weight loss. Eventually, however, you notice that you've reached a plateau. You cannot understand how exerting more effort and eating less is causing weight gain rather than weight loss. You stick it out for a short time longer but eventually give up your exercise program, wondering what happened.

  Had you followed your physician's instructions and consulted her before dramatically increasing the time and speed of your workout or altering the diet, you would have learned that (1) the level of extended exertion was actually traumatizing your body and one of the effects is a tendency to gain weight (this is an effect of the hormone cortisol and other bodily reactions); (2) your metabolism slows as you age; (3) the paradoxical negative impact of eliminating carbs from your diet; (4) underestimation of the number of calories in certain foods; and (5) a tendency to gain weight due to sleep deprivation. This is a situation in which a lack of accurate information led to failure. Besides, if you had viewed the exercise and diet regimen as action steps in an overall health/fitness goal, the weight loss issue would not have been seen as the sole indicator of success or failure.

- One of my coaching clients, a senior executive in his organization, reported that he became quite anxious prior to giving presentations in front of large groups. Over the years, he had worked around this problem in various ways, such as having the presentation given by a subordinate and calling in to participate via teleconference. Helping clients become confident and skilled presenters is well within the scope of a coaching engagement and an issue with which I had broad experience. I was ready to roll up my sleeves and have my client and I dive in together to solve his problem. However, during the discovery process it became clear that the root of his anxiety was much deeper and more pronounced. Before we could proceed, my client had to address the psychological issues that were contributing to his anxiety.

7. Values Conflict

Conflict in values is perhaps the most overlooked barrier by change agents. If a goal, or an action step to reach your goal, no matter how reasonably thought out and researched, is in conflict with a closely-held value, frustration with the conflict will eventually derail your plan.

- A client of mine had begun a new weight-loss plan. After a couple of weeks, she reverted to eating the same foods that she served her children. Upon questioning, she informed me that the only quality time she had with her kids was during dinner. It frustrated her that her new meal plan required her to first cook the children's dinner and, while they were eating, to fix hers. My response, "Family is really important to you, isn't it?" "Oh, absolutely, it's more important to me than anything else," she replied. I then congratulated her on failing to honor her previous commitment to cook special meals for herself. Why did I honor her? Because even though health is very important to her, by cooking separate meals she was missing out on quality time with her kids and thus dishonoring a higher value—family.

  Had she been aware of a potential conflict, she could have avoided this pitfall by working out a plan that would allow her to both join her children at dinner and lose weight. After discussing her options, she agreed to focus her dieting around breakfast, lunch, and any meals outside the home. In addition, she committed to a 20-minute walk with the children after dinner. This would allow her to work off any excess calories she may have consumed during dinner and have some additional kid time.

- From a business standpoint, a values conflict could mean misaligned incentives. For example, I once worked with the partners of a law firm who were attempting to create a more cooperative environment, yet their compensation schedule was based on individual performance. In addition to clearly identifying a business strategy, they needed to also make changes to their compensation structure. Other examples I have seen in my work as an executive coach include: a workplace that allegedly encourages a healthy work-life balance but rewards employees who arrive early and stay late; and a company that publicizes its focus on a healthy lifestyle but celebrates all occasions of corporate and individual success with "happy hours." When values at work conflict, it can result in frustration and anger among staff members and, in the extreme, create a hostile work environment.

A certain company that has successfully instituted a number of innovative workplace programs encourages open dialogue among, and buy-in from, the entire workforce. They have an employee-management committee which thoroughly researches all sides of an issue, ensuring that there are no conflicts in corporate vs. staff values. Recommendations are mutually developed and submitted for corporate review. When approved, the committee helps implement the plan and regularly evaluates it for any needed correction or modification.

If values conflict is negatively affecting your entire workplace, perhaps you can encourage your coworkers to mobilize and suggest a similar plan to management. If the values conflict affects only you, it will be necessary to look carefully at the impact it is having on your life. Here, again, take advantage of resources within your Human Resources department (EAP, Executive Coach) to aid in your resolution of the situation. After weighing possible options, you will be able to determine if continued employment with this company is in your best interest.

Chapter 5

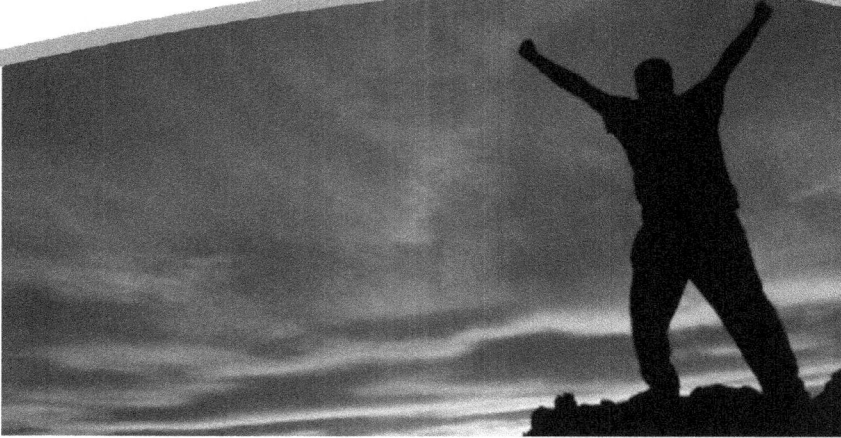

INTO ACTION

*"Your life will be no better than
the plans you make and the action you take.
You are the architect and builder of
your own life, fortune, destiny."*
Alfred A. Montapert, 1906-1997

FOUR STEPS TO SUSTAINED CHANGE

In the previous chapters, you learned why willpower doesn't work in creating and sustaining habit change; the importance of bringing into awareness, and owning, your subconscious actions; the seven action steps to prepare for change; and the seven common barriers to change and how to overcome them.

In this chapter we will discuss the steps necessary to sustain change. The mindfulness practices are described in detail. You will have an opportunity to ensure that your intention, goal, action steps, and measurement factors are all in sync.

MEDITATE
--> Set intention and goal
--> Take action
--> Overcome barriers

MINDFULNESS MEDITATION PRACTICE

To develop a practice of meditation, commit to just 2-5 minutes per day. It helps to find the same time each day, such as shortly after awakening—perhaps after a shower but before you begin your workday, or in the early evening, such as before dinner or bedtime. If you meditate towards bedtime and find yourself falling asleep during the meditation, it could mean you are not getting enough sleep at night. Try to improve your sleep habits and/or meditate earlier in the day. There are websites and apps for your Smartphone that you may find helpful in leading you through your meditation. Following are some general guidelines:

1. Sit with your back and neck straight in a comfortable, quiet environment, with soft lighting. Wear comfortable clothing. Remain as still as possible.

2. With eyes and mouth closed, breathe through your nose. Let the breath flow naturally. Become aware of the beginning, middle, and end of each breath. When distractions arise, gently but firmly bring your attention back to the breath.

3. Notice without judgment the thoughts, images, sensations, and feelings that surface in your mind, while focusing on your breath or some other object of awareness, such as a mantra—a word or phrase which you silently repeat with each breath.

4. As thoughts, images, sensations, and feelings arise, pay "bare attention" to them. Observe the tendency to hold on to pleasant thoughts, images, sensations, and feelings and to push away unpleasant ones. Observe but do not label a thought as "good" or "bad." Become aware of the impermanent nature of all thoughts, images, sensations, and feelings.

By cultivating this disciplined mind, you break down the illusion within your mind of who you are, leading to greater self-awareness. In a more practical sense, you train the mind to work for you by helping you live a happier and healthier life, rather than working against you by getting caught up in judgments that can lead to anxiety, depression and poor health.

THE THREE QUESTION MANTRA

As you learned in Chapter 2, the three question mantra is another mindfulness process that will help you adhere to your action plan. *"Mantra", as used here, simply refers to a message that you repeatedly tell yourself.* Not to be confused with a meditation mantra, the three question mantra is used throughout the day to help with decision-making. I refer to it as a mantra because the intention is for it to be used often, so much so that its repetition is like that of a meditation mantra, silently repeated over and over.

The questions you choose for your mantra should relate

specifically to your goal. In the example below, the goal is good health, so the first two questions relate to good health. You will substitute your own word or phrase, depending on your goal. Keep the questions at the forefront of your mind so that each time you're confronted with a decision, they'll be immediately accessible.

Example: Assume that you have been diagnosed with heart disease and your goal is to significantly improve your health. This is how the in-the-moment accountability structure would work for you:

You are faced with a choice—fruit or cake. Prior to taking action, you ask yourself the following question:

1. Do I want health or do I not want health?

If the answer is "I don't want health," then the process is done for that moment and you will make your choice, likely the unhealthy one. In a sense, the concern is not whether you make the healthy versus unhealthy choice. The key is that you make a conscious choice. In fact, in teaching this method to clients, I stress the importance of avoiding shame over making the unhealthy choice. This is not about "making one choose health over non-health," nor is it about shaming one for choosing non-health. Instead, it is about putting a wedge of awareness between a thought and an action. It helps you step back for the moment and remind yourself of your goal which, in this case, is to be healthy.

If you choose health, ask yourself the second question:

2. Do I choose health right now or do I choose non-health right now?

Notice the first question is global and is derived from your goal – to be healthy. The answer to the first question will almost always be "Yes" if the goal and associated mantra were chosen carefully. The second question moves you to a "right now decision." It asks you to consciously support or sabotage your goal. Two key words in the second question are, "choose," and "now." Similar to the well-known Alcoholics Anonymous mantra, "One day at a time," referring to the choice not to drink for that day versus committing to never drinking again, this second question and the whole process is about making choices one moment at a time. If you decide to "choose non-health now," the process is done for that moment and you will make your choice, likely the unhealthy one.

If you choose "health now," ask yourself the third and final question:

3. What action do I need to take right now?

The decision has been made and you act in accordance with your conscious choice. In this case, it would be to choose the fruit over the cake. The "action" could also be to avoid something, such as to avoid a second helping of dessert.

Important Considerations:

- The first question is always structured as the desire (e.g., health) followed by "non-desire" (e.g., non-health). While it may be tempting to make the second choice a variation of its opposite, such as "disease" or "poor health," in this case, doing so will almost always be inherently biased and could lead to mixed results. For example, substituting "disease" for non-health could lead you to doubt the outcome ("Am I really going to get a disease if I have this one piece of cake?") and thus doubt the process.

- The phrasing of the second question is also important. Notice that "...or do I choose non-health now?" is different than "Do I choose health now or not now." In the former, the emphasis of "not" is on choosing health, whereas in the latter the emphasis is on "now," which could suggest that you can have the cake now and health later.

- The third question is always the same and independent of the goal.

- It is important to keep the questions and the process simple.

- It is also imperative to avoid shaming judgment, keeping in mind the purpose is to raise awareness. Even if you make mostly poor decisions initially, this is likely to improve over time.

This method of in-the-moment accountability helps raise awareness over choices that might otherwise be made without conscious thought. The entire process takes about 10 seconds.

As noted above, but worth repeating: the three question mantra is most powerful when used throughout the day. An easy way to cultivate its practice is to begin by saying it to yourself at the beginning of your day, such as when brushing your teeth or showering, and whenever it comes to mind throughout the day. The more often you repeat it, the greater will be the chance that you'll remember it when you're about to make a decision—such as choosing a dessert—that will either support of hinder achievement of your goal.

Once you become comfortable with the three question mantra, you may find yourself using it frequently throughout the day, in any number of situations. The following examples focus only on the second question:

Do I choose to be on time (right now)?
Or do I choose to not be on time (right now)?

Do I choose to eat healthy (right now)?
Or do I choose to not eat healthy (right now)?

Do I choose to leave the house in a good frame of mind (right now)?
Or do I choose to leave the house not in a good frame of mind (right now)?

Do I choose to be productive (right now)?
Or do I choose to not be productive (right now)?

Do I choose to be creative (right now)?
Or do I choose not to be creative (right now)?

Do I choose to support getting eight hours of sleep (right now)?
Or do I choose not to support getting eight hours of sleep (right now)?

As you can see, the list is as endless as your decisions. The questions become easy to generate with a little practice and grow to be second nature with a bit more practice.

In the coaching environment, this process can be used by a coach whenever a client is wavering on a commitment. Asking these questions shifts the accountability back to the client, where it belongs.

Meditate
    --> SET INTENTION AND GOAL
      --> Take action
        --> Overcome barriers

SET AN INTENTION.

An intention is different from a goal. A goal is a target you work to achieve and measure through an action plan. An intention is a higher conscious thought. It sets your "aim" without placing restrictions on the "how" or process of achieving the desire. An intention is not measured by success or failure.

I intend to be at my ideal weight.

I intend to be highly successful at work.

I intend to be exceptionally compassionate towards others.

EXERCISE

Set a clear intention. Be sure your intention is concise and as simply presented as possible.

SET A GOAL.

A goal captures your intention and makes it actionable. Examples of achievable goals using the intentions above are:

My goal is to lose 10 pounds before June 1st.

My goal is to receive two promotions before the end of the year, doubling my current salary and increasing my responsibilities by 50%.

My goal is to act and speak in ways which support others' best interest and never self-promote at others' expense.

EXERCISE

Identify a goal. Make it R.E.A.L.

REALISTIC

Given your life circumstances, is the goal itself *and* are the action steps to accomplish it realistic (e.g., lose 20 pounds before December 31 by eating less than 11,200 calories per week and getting at least 7 hours of sleep for at least 4 days per week throughout the remainder of the year)?

EVALUATIVE

Will I know when I've achieved my goal? Can I measure the goal? If two different people were assessing my success or failure would they see the same thing (e.g., "walking 5 minutes per day, 3 days per week for 15 weeks" versus "walk more" or "walk 3 times per week")?

Meditate
--> Set intention and goal
--> TAKE ACTION
--> Overcome barriers

DEVELOP AN ACTION PLAN.

Change happens only when you take action. However, efforts to initiate change often fail because people too often jump into action without raising their awareness, setting a clear intent, and defining a R.E.A.L. goal.

An effective action plan is one that, if properly executed, will help you achieve your goal. An action plan can be developed at once or in increments. For example, if your goal is to lose 15 pounds in 12 weeks, your action plan might be as follows:

1. Go to bed before 10 PM at least 4 days per week. Plan to do so for the next 12 weeks but reevaluate after 2 weeks.

2. Count calories each day: consume no more than 11,200 calories per week, averaging 1,600 calories per day, for the next 2 weeks; re-evaluate after 2 weeks.

3. Perform 20 minutes of interval training on the elliptical at least 3 times per week. Plan to do so for the next 12 weeks but reevaluate after 2 weeks.

4. Check weight every Thursday morning upon waking for the next 12 weeks.

5. Meditate 2-5 minutes per day, 5 days per week. Plan to do so for the next 12 weeks but reevaluate after 2 weeks.

Notice how every item except number 4 (Check weight every Thursday morning upon waking for the next 12 weeks) provides a starting point, an end point, and a reevaluation point. The advantage is that it allows for adjustments to the plan along the way should anything unexpected occur. Creating sustained change for more than 2 weeks at a time (unless you're a pro) can be very difficult unless the change is relatively easy to do without making significant sacrifice (such as in number 4). I highly recommend that you commit to your action plan for no more than two weeks at a time.

TRACK YOUR PROGRESS.

It is highly recommended that you create a simple chart to track your success.

REWARD SUCCESS.

It is important to reward success. Often clients tell me achieving the desired goal is reward enough but, if that were true, they would already have achieved their goal.

Reward successful actions, not outcomes. In the above example, I would recommend that you reward yourself at the end of each week for completing each of the five action steps. Reward should be an incentive but also realistic. It can be as simple as treating oneself to a movie. Rewards ideally should "fit the goal" and not work against the goal. For example, instead of rewarding yourself with binge eating on Sunday for completing all action steps Monday through Saturday (thus undoing much of your great effort), consider putting $20 per successful week in a fund to purchase new clothes at the end of the 12 weeks.

Notice that the $20 per week you are creating is a "token reward" that increases in value over time. This is an excellent way to reward weekly success while building a greater and more significant reward for total success. If using a token reward system, it is okay to have the end reward linked to the outcome (e.g., losing 15 pounds) but be cautious with this. Failing to achieve your desired goal may be due to events beyond your control, and you do not want to punish yourself for circumstances over which you have no influence.

A way to significantly step up your action plan and increase the likelihood of success is to identify consequences for each action item when developing your plan. Too often people make a commitment, e.g., to exercise 3 times per week, only to miss a day and then to give up on the entire plan. This happens because a failure response is triggered and the sacrifices required to achieve the goal no longer seem worth the effort. There is a shift from seeing oneself as successful to accepting failure. By setting out consequences, you get ahead of this challenge and build success into the program.

KEEP THE PLAN IN EFFECT AND FUNCTIONING

ACTION: Go to bed before 10 PM at least 4 days per week for the next 2 weeks; reevaluate.

CONSEQUENCE: (for not getting to bed before 10 PM for at least 4 days in a given week): Forgo watching any television after 6 PM the entire next week (this assumes that watching television in the evening is a regular and enjoyable activity). This consequence is especially fitting if the main barrier to getting to bed on time is watching television past 10 PM.

ACTION: Count calories each day and eat no more than 11,200 calories per week, averaging 1,600 calories per day, for the next 2 weeks; re-evaluate.

CONSEQUENCE: (for eating more than 11,200 calories in a given week): Abstain from eating refined sugar or drinking alcoholic beverages and soda for one week, starting the day after exceeding 11,200 calories within a period of one week.

ACTION: Do 20 minutes of interval training on the elliptical at least 3 times per week for the next 2 weeks; re-evaluate.

CONSEQUENCE: (for doing the elliptical less than 60 minutes over 3 days in a given week): Make up for lost time the following week by increasing the number of minutes on any given day and/or add more days (e.g., 4 days instead of 3).

ACTION: Weigh self every Thursday morning upon waking for the next 12 weeks.

CONSEQUENCE: (for weighing self on a day other than Thursday or not weighing self on Thursday): NONE.

ACTION: Meditate 5 minutes per day, 5 days per week for the next 2 weeks; re-evaluate.

CONSEQUENCE: (for meditating less than 5 minutes and/or less than 5 times in a given week): Increase meditation time to 10 minutes per day over 5 days in the following week.

Notice how the action step of weighing oneself does not have an associated consequence. This is because the action step is a support structure but does not have a direct impact on reaching the goal.

Also notice how the consequences "fit the crime" and are uncomfortable but not unrealistic. It is important to select the consequence carefully so it falls within an acceptable range of but is not overwhelming. I have found that setting up a restriction such as "No refined sugar or white flour for 12 weeks" sets off the rebel within us that does not like to be told "No" and, rather than being successful, we challenge the restriction, which sets off the failure response. Instead, setting a consequence such as, "If I eat refined sugar or white flour, I must reduce my allowable caloric intake by 500 calories the following week," specifies something to avoid rather than something to challenge.

Notice too that one will likely achieve the same outcome regardless of whether or not he abides by the defined action step (No refined sugar or white flour) or its consequence (reduce caloric intake by 500 calories the following week).

ACTION-ORIENTED

Does your goal lead to clear action steps? For example, "Smoke one less cigarette per week and take three deep breaths before each cigarette" versus "quit smoking."

LIMITED

Is your goal time-limited, recognizing that success breeds success. For example, "Meditate for 5 minutes each day for 2 weeks" versus "Meditate 5 minutes each day."

Gathering the correct information and defining R.E.A.L. goals and action steps may help you achieve your goal when you are otherwise feeling confused.

EXERCISE

Identify a goal. Make sure it is R.E.A.L.

R = Realistic: Is it possible to achieve the goal given your timeline and your current situation?

E = Evaluative: Can you easily measure your goal?

A = Action-oriented: Does your goal easily lead to specific actions that you can take to achieve it?

L = Time-limited: Does your goal (and associated action steps) have a very specific timeframe for achieving it?

Meditate
--> Set intention and goal
--> Take action
--> OVERCOME BARRIERS

Attempting to create a significant change will almost inevitably lead to self-sabotaging behavior. In the next section we will revisit the Barriers to Change and introduce ways to identify and overcome each barrier.

OVERCOMING BARRIERS

Be sure you have reviewed the seven common barriers outlined in Chapter 4. You will recall they are likely to surface when you put your plan into action. You will empower your ability to create sustained change by meeting the inevitable roadblocks with specific solutions. These tools to overcoming barriers are the same "inside secrets" used in a 126-hour coach training program I co-developed to train coaches to be effective in helping clients change their behavior.

1. Obtain accurate information.

2. Clearly identify a specific and measurable goal.

3. Select only goals for which you are truly motivated, realizing "small" is better.

4. Start with small, easy-to-achieve steps, building confidence over time.

5. Acquire the necessary resources and support to help you succeed.

6. Address medical or psychological issues with your healthcare providers.

7. Be sure your goal and method of reaching it are aligned with your values.

Consider using the following acronym
to help you design a successful habit change plan:

IMAGES

I: Right Information & Right Intention

M: Right Mind (mindful, motivated, confident)

A: Right Action (small steps, clearly defined, action-focused)

G: Right Goal (R.E.A.L.)

E: Right Environment (structural/environmental modification)

S: Right Support (nonjudgmental, objective, supportive)

SUPPORT RESOURCES

For assistance in acheiving your habit change goals:

1-on-1 coaching or group classes, visit my website:
www.drjeffkaplan.com

Further information and support services, send email to:
drjeff@drjeffkaplan.com

Jeff Kaplan, Ph.D.

ABOUT THE AUTHOR

This book was written to share with readers the experience and insights Dr. Kaplan has acquired over his 30 years of research and practice in helping people create sustained change.

Dr. Kaplan began his helping career at age 20, while still in college, working primarily with adjudicated youth, but gradually increasing his focus to children across the spectrum—from those with autism to violent offenders. His early clients were found in hospitals, detention centers, schools, residential institutions, and on the streets (working with runaway youth).

In the early 1990's, while obtaining his doctorate in psychology, Dr. Kaplan's career began to shift as he was called upon to create change programs on various aspects of health. In 1995, he was invited to join a team of consultants to assist the senior executives of a large company understand the cause of, and to resolve, the interpersonal conflicts within their organization. In the late 1990's Dr. Kaplan received training as a professional coach and has been providing coaching, training and consulting ever since. In 2005, he received his Masters in Business Administration and co-founded, with Steve Baumgartner and Dr. Bob Bulgarelli, the Habit Change Company. As Chief Operating Officer, he designs programs to support individuals and organizations create and maintain healthful habits and practices.

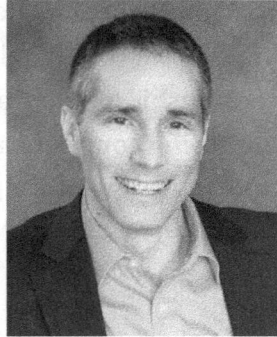

Today, Dr. Kaplan continues to develop and facilitate innovative habit change programs and helps train coaches throughout the country to do the same. He also consults with organizations, designs and delivers training programs, and provides executive coaching to senior and emerging leaders, all with a focus on changing behavior as it relates to almost all aspects of interpersonal relationships. Such areas of focus include: influencing others, improving communication, developing and motivating employees, understanding office politics, increasing confidence and executive presence, resolving conflict, and becoming a more mindful leader.

ACKNOWLEDGEMENT

First and foremost, I would like to acknowledge my mother, Pat Gallagher. Her, response to, "Hey, Mom, can you take a quick look at this and check for any grammatical or spelling errors," led to many early mornings, late evenings and, (dare I say) 3 A.M. bedtimes. Her editing, restructuring, adding and clarifying the content of this book is what made it easily digestible for the typical reader. Her approach to helping me with this book is a perfect demonstration of one of the important values she taught me growing up, which is to always "go above and beyond". I thank you, Mom, for instilling in me a sense of work excellence and professionalism.

I'd also like to thank my wonderful sister, Debbie Kaplan, who also spent many hours, including days off from work, editing and improving the early and final drafts. In addition, I am grateful to my friend and colleague, Ryan Wexelblatt, who provided great production assistance and graciously put up with many "final versions" after already starting the production process. Thanks also to Lorie DeWorken who provided her expertise in the areas of design and formatting.

Finally, I'd like to acknowledge my life partner, Matt Ochs, for his constant love and support. I love you — yesterday, today, tomorrow, always, forever and beyond.